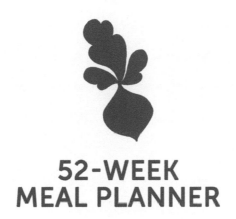

52-WEEK
MEAL PLANNER

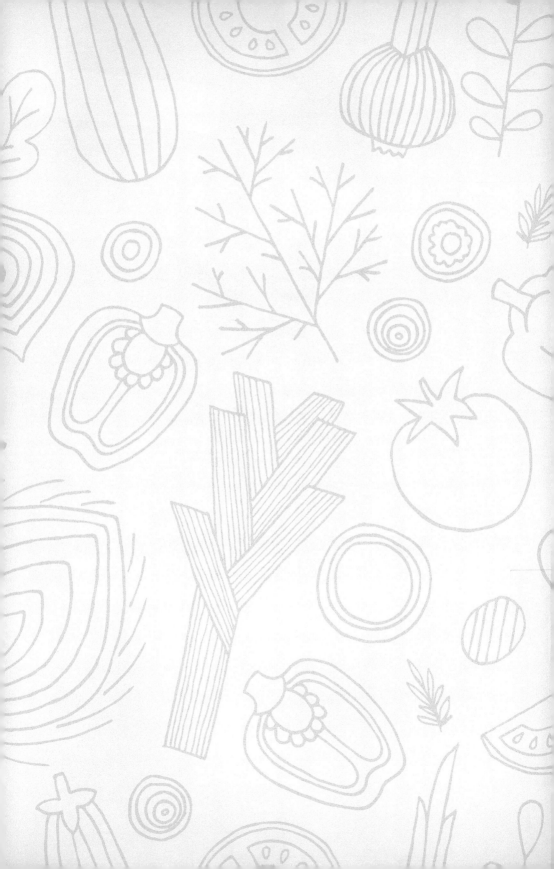

52 WEEK
MEAL PLANNER

The Complete Guide
to Planning Menus,
Groceries, Recipes,
and More

JESSICA LEVINSON, MS, RDN, CDN

ROCKRIDGE
PRESS

For general information on our other products and services or to obtain technical support, please contact our Customer Care Department within the United States at (866) 744-2665, or outside the United States at (510) 253-0500.

Rockridge Press publishes its books in a variety of electronic and print formats. Some content that appears in print may not be available in electronic books, and vice versa.

Designer: Christopher T. Fong
Editor: Meg Ilasco
Production Editor: Andrew Yackira
Illustrations © Adehoidar / iStock, 2017

ISBN: Print 978-1-64152-156-7

CONTENTS

Introduction   7

Best Practices for Balancing Meals   8
Best Practices for Feeding a Family   10
Meal Prep Hacks   11
How to Use This Weekly Meal Planner   12
Seasonal Produce Guide   14

Weekly Meal Planner   20
Recipe Pages   130
Price Comparisons   146
Weekly Shopping Lists   161

INTRODUCTION

IT'S 5:00 PM, you're standing at the refrigerator peering inside to see what's on hand for dinner, the kids are clamoring for something to eat, and you're ready to call for takeout, again.

Or perhaps you live alone and you've come home after a long day of work, ready to put your feet up, veg out in front of the TV, and eat your dinner, only to find there's nothing in your fridge or freezer.

Sound familiar? You're not alone. According to a 2017 consumer survey, almost half of Americans eat a home-cooked meal less than twice a week, and in fact, most of the people who rely on takeout weren't planning to.[1]

Whether you're trying to feed a family, eat healthier, reduce food waste, or save money and time, meal planning is a lifestyle habit that can help you achieve these goals. In fact, meal planning is a smart way to get healthy, balanced meals on the table for yourself and your family throughout the week—and it takes less effort than you might think.

The best strategy to ensure you follow a meal plan is to write it down. This workbook will help you get organized and stay organized as you get in the swing of planning your weekly meals and grocery trips. You'll have a place to record your favorite recipes and compare prices of your frequently purchased ingredients. To help with meal inspiration and money savings, I've also included best practices for balancing meals, meal prep hacks, and a seasonal produce guide. Planning meals has never been easier!

---

1   Hartman Group. *Transformation of the American Meal*, 2017.

BEST PRACTICES FOR BALANCING MEALS

One of the greatest benefits of meal planning is that it leads to healthier eating habits. Thinking through what you're serving ahead of time allows you to plan out balanced meals throughout the day and week. Sure, some people could plan a week of unhealthy meals, but most people who meal plan do so with a healthy, balanced diet in mind. What does that entail?

A balanced diet is composed of fruits, vegetables, protein, healthy oils, grains, and low- and nonfat dairy. It's also one that limits saturated and trans fats, added sugar, and sodium. How these food groups come together on your plate can vary endlessly from meal to meal, but on a daily basis, it is recommended that an adult on a 2,000-calorie diet consume the following:

FRUIT: 2-cup equivalent

1-cup equivalent: 1 cup sliced fruit, 1 cup 100% fruit juice, ½ cup dried fruit

VEGETABLES: 2½-cup equivalent

1-cup equivalent: 1 cup raw or cooked vegetables, 1 cup 100% vegetable juice, 2 cups leafy salad greens

Examples: dark green vegetables (such as leafy greens, broccoli); red and orange vegetables (such as carrots, peppers, tomatoes, sweet potatoes); legumes (such as beans, split peas, edamame); starchy vegetables (such as potatoes, corn, green peas)

LEAN PROTEIN: 5½-ounce equivalent

1-ounce equivalent: 1 ounce lean meat, poultry, or seafood, 1 egg, ¼ cup cooked beans or tofu, 1 tablespoon nut butter, ½ ounce nuts or seeds

Examples: skinless chicken breast, 90% lean ground beef, lamb, eggs, fish and seafood

HEALTHY OILS: 27 grams (about 2 tablespoons)

Examples: canola, corn, olive, peanut, safflower, soybean, and sunflower

GRAINS: 6-ounce equivalent, with at least half whole grains

1-ounce equivalent: ½ cup cooked rice, pasta, or cereal; 1 ounce sliced bread; 1 cup ready-to-eat cereal

Examples of whole grains: whole-wheat bread, oatmeal, quinoa, popcorn, brown rice

DAIRY: 3-cup equivalents

1-cup equivalent: 1 cup low-fat or nonfat milk or yogurt, 1 cup fortified soy beverage, 1½ ounces natural cheese (such as Cheddar or Swiss), ⅓ cup shredded cheese, 2 cups cottage cheese

As you consider how to portion these food groups throughout the day, keep in mind the image of a balanced plate: half the plate filled with vegetables and fruit, one-quarter of the plate filled with whole grains, and the remaining quarter of the plate filled with lean protein. Healthy oils and low-fat and nonfat dairy foods should be dispersed throughout the day, and water—even naturally flavored—is always the beverage of choice.

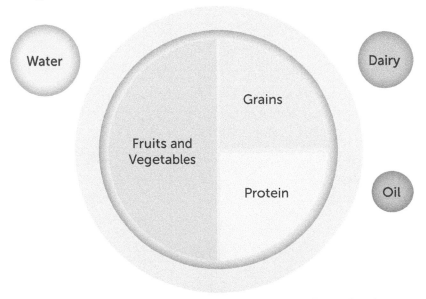

BEST PRACTICES FOR FEEDING A FAMILY

Feeding a family is no easy task, but having a plan of action can make it so much easier. Time is *always* of the essence when kids are involved, and planning is the number-one way to ensure that tasks get done in a way you can feel good about. Here are six best practices for feeding a family:

Map out your menu on paper. The act of writing down your menu helps you visualize your plan, holds you accountable to it, and helps you remember what's on tap for the week as you look ahead. Most importantly, it helps you stay on track with meal prep.

Generate a shopping list. Once your menu is in place, put pen to paper (or fingers to smartphone) and make your grocery list for the week. Include perishable items you need specifically for this week's meals, nonperishable staples you need to replenish, and any additional items, based on what's on sale or family requests.

Keep a well-stocked kitchen. There are certain staples everyone should have on hand, such as healthy oils, whole grains, canned foods, dried herbs and spices, low-sodium broth, and nuts and seeds. The same goes for the refrigerator and freezer—low-fat plain and Greek yogurt, frozen corn, eggs, low-fat cheeses, and fruit and vegetables are just some examples. You'll save time and money and reduce food waste by basing your meal plans around those staples. Sometimes the most family-friendly meals are the ones put together from what's already available at home—think homemade mac and cheese, casseroles, chili, frittatas, yogurt parfaits—all easy to throw together with ingredients at arm's reach.

Make meal planning and prep a family affair. When kids are involved in deciding what they're eating and cooking it, they are more likely to eat what's served.

Plan theme nights. Meatless Monday, Taco Tuesday, Wacky Wednesday, Fish Friday . . . you get the idea. Kids love when there's a theme to dinner, and it makes planning the menu easier because you know exactly what kind of recipe you need for every night of the week.

Don't be a short-order cook. Instead, make one meal for the whole family and ensure there is at least one item on the table that each person likes. Serving meals buffet-style or like a "bar" is a fun way to make one meal while still allowing for personal choice.

MEAL PREP HACKS

Meal planning is the first step in getting healthy meals on the table. Meal prep is the second, and that's where most of the time and work come in. However, you can make meal prep faster and easier with these eight tips:

1. **Ease into meal prep.** Start with recipes that don't require too many ingredients or a lot of hands-on time.

2. **Prep several recipes worth of produce.** Wash, peel, chop, zest, or juice all your fruits and vegetables at once. For the freshest produce, plan to do this at least twice during each week.

3. **Roast an assortment of vegetables.** These can be used for various meals throughout the week—add them to salads, fold into frittatas, toss into pasta dishes, or simply serve as a side dish.

4. **Prepare multiple things at once.** To make the most of your time, you can marinate chicken, cook a batch of quinoa, and chop vegetables all at the same time.

5. **Start prepping what takes the longest first.** For example, get your soup in the slow cooker before you make your salad.

6. **Double or triple recipes.** This will ensure you have healthy meals on hand for days when you don't have time to cook. Soups and stews, casseroles, burgers, egg frittatas, and muffins all freeze well and are not too much extra work to double. Even whole grains freeze well and can easily be used as the base of a future lunch or dinner.

7. **Stock up on certain convenience foods.** Good options for saving time prepping on busy nights include stir-in herb and spice pastes, microwaveable whole grains, shredded cabbage and Brussels sprouts, prechopped vegetables like mirepoix (onions, celery, and carrots), butternut squash, and broccoli florets.

8. **Label your prep work.** Do this before you put it in the refrigerator or freezer, so you don't one day find yourself staring at five bags of frozen sauce, unable to remember if they are Bolognese or fra diavolo. There's nothing worse than taking the time to prep in advance, only to forget what you have on hand, especially when it's 30 minutes before dinnertime!

HOW TO USE THIS WEEKLY MEAL PLANNER

Now that you have an idea of what you and your family need to eat for a balanced meal and some of the best tips for making these meals happen, it's time for you to start meal planning. The pages of this meal planning workbook contain templates for your weekly meal plan, recipe pages, note sections, price comparison sheets, and blank shopping lists. In short, you have everything you need to make these healthy, balanced meals happen!

It may seem pretty intuitive how to go about using the elements of the meal planner, but read on for some tips on the best way to put this book to use.

WEEKLY MEAL PLANNER

Each weekly meal planner is a two-page spread that has room for you to write down breakfast, lunch, dinner, and snacks for the day. When filling in the planner, be as specific as possible and list side dishes in addition to mains. When listing your snack for the day, keep in mind that some people only eat one snack a day, whereas others eat two (or more).

If you're not quite ready to plan out the whole week, don't stress. The key to sticking to goals is to start small and build on success. Ease into meal planning by planning two days of the week or one meal a day for the first couple of weeks. Note that there are 55 planners included, in case you make a mistake and need to start over. If you need recipe ideas for your weekly meal plan, go to the "Recipe Library" at JessicaLevinson.com.

The notes section at the end of each weekly meal planner is the perfect place to jot down reminders of ingredients you need for that specific week, note if someone is out one night, or calculate how much of a certain ingredient you need, which will help you organize your shopping list.

RECIPE PAGES

The recipe pages included in the planner are perfect for writing down your favorite, go-to recipes. These may be the recipes that are in your meal plan every week or ones you batch cook once a month.

PRICE COMPARISONS

One of the benefits of meal planning is that it can save you money by only purchasing what you need and by basing your plan on the price of groceries and what's on sale. Use the price comparison worksheets to compare prices at different stores for groceries you often purchase and sale items every week. You can then use the comparison sheet to make your shopping lists according to store.

SHOPPING LIST

One of the best practices for feeding a family is making a shopping list to go along with your meal plan. The list keeps you on track to buy only what you need, which saves you time and money. Use the shopping lists at the end of the book to organize your grocery list by store. Cut each list out with scissors and use one list per shopping trip. It's also efficient to organize the list by the layout of the store. For example, most supermarkets open into the produce section, so start the list with all your fruits and vegetables for the week, with inner-aisle items grouped together further down on the list.

SEASONAL PRODUCE GUIDE

SPRING	SUMMER
Apples	Apples
Apricots	Apricots
Asparagus	Avocado
Avocado	Bananas
Bananas	Beets
Broccoli	Bell Peppers
Cabbage	Blackberries
Carrots	Blueberries
Celery	Carrots
Collard Greens	Cantaloupe/Muskmelons
Garlic	Celery
Greens (cooking)	Cherries
Lettuce	Collard Greens
Mushrooms	Corn
Onions	Cucumbers
Peas	Eggplant
Pineapple	Garlic
Radishes	Green Beans
Rhubarb	Honeydew Melon
Spinach	Kiwifruit
Strawberries	Lima Beans
Swiss Chard	Mangos
Turnips	Nectarines
	Okra
	Peaches
	Plums
	Raspberries
	Strawberries
	Summer Squash & Zucchini
	Tomatillos
	Tomatoes
	Watermelon

Source: United States Department of Agriculture (USDA)

FALL	WINTER
Apples	Apples
Bananas	Avocado
Beets	Bananas
Bell Peppers	Beets
Broccoli	Brussels Sprouts
Brussels Sprouts	Cabbage
Cabbage	Carrots
Carrots	Celery
Cauliflower	Grapefruit
Celery	Kale
Collard Greens	Leeks
Cranberries	Lemons
Garlic	Onions
Ginger	Oranges
Grapes	Parsnips
Greens (cooking)	Pears
Green Beans	Pineapple
Kale	Potatoes
Lettuce	Pumpkins
Mangos	Rutabagas
Mushrooms	Sweet Potatoes and Yams
Onions	Turnips
Parsnips	Winter Squash
Peas	
Pears	
Pineapple	
Potatoes	
Pumpkins	
Radishes	
Raspberries	
Rutabagas	
Spinach	
Sweet Potatoes and Yams	
Swiss Chard	
Turnips	
Winter Squash	

WEEKLY MEAL PLANNER

MONDAY

	BREAKFAST	LUNCH	DINNER
	Bran flakes, strawberries, skim milk	Tuna sandwich on whole-wheat bread, sliced cucumbers and tomatoes, grapes	Crispy baked tofu with roasted sweet potatoes and carrots, brown rice

SNACK: Yogurt and granola

TUESDAY

	BREAKFAST	LUNCH	DINNER
	Cottage cheese, cereal and berries	Salad with leftover roasted veggies and tofu from Mon. night dinner	Panko chicken, roasted Brussels sprouts, and quinoa salad

SNACK: Roasted chickpeas and apple

WEDNESDAY

	BREAKFAST	LUNCH	DINNER
	Mixed berry smoothie	Avocado toast and side salad	Mediterranean Sheet Pan Salmon with Zucchini, Corn and Tomatoes

SNACK: Veggies and hummus

THURSDAY

	BREAKFAST	LUNCH	DINNER
	Peaches and cream Overnight Oats	Greek salad with grilled chicken	Mushroom onion frittata, side salad, and whole grain sourdough toast

SNACK: Apple and peanut butter

	BREAKFAST	LUNCH	DINNER
FRIDAY	Yogurt, berries, and granola	Leftover frittata and salad	Make your own pizza night!

SNACK: Popcorn trail mix

	BREAKFAST	LUNCH	DINNER
SATURDAY	Baked French Toast and mixed berries	Assorted leftovers from the week	Night out!

SNACK: Nuts and dried fruit

	BREAKFAST	LUNCH	DINNER
SUNDAY	Scrambled eggs, whole-wheat toast, grapefruit	Chicken salad sandwiches and side salad	Lightened Up Macaroni and Cheese and roasted broccoli

SNACK: Frozen yogurt pop

NOTES & CALCULATIONS

Thursday — Joe is out for dinner
Sunday — double dinner — Kate's friends coming over

WEEKLY
MEAL
PLANNER

Weekly Meal Planner   20
Recipe Pages   130
Price Comparisons   146
Weekly Shopping List   161

	BREAKFAST	LUNCH	DINNER
MONDAY			

SNACK:

	BREAKFAST	LUNCH	DINNER
TUESDAY			

SNACK:

	BREAKFAST	LUNCH	DINNER
WEDNESDAY			

SNACK:

	BREAKFAST	LUNCH	DINNER
THURSDAY			

SNACK:

	BREAKFAST	LUNCH	DINNER
FRIDAY			

SNACK:

	BREAKFAST	LUNCH	DINNER
SATURDAY			

SNACK:

	BREAKFAST	LUNCH	DINNER
SUNDAY			

SNACK:

NOTES & CALCULATIONS

WEEKLY MEAL PLANNER

	BREAKFAST	LUNCH	DINNER
MONDAY			

SNACK:

	BREAKFAST	LUNCH	DINNER
TUESDAY			

SNACK:

	BREAKFAST	LUNCH	DINNER
WEDNESDAY			

SNACK:

	BREAKFAST	LUNCH	DINNER
THURSDAY			

SNACK:

	BREAKFAST	LUNCH	DINNER
FRIDAY			

SNACK:

	BREAKFAST	LUNCH	DINNER
SATURDAY			

SNACK:

	BREAKFAST	LUNCH	DINNER
SUNDAY			

SNACK:

NOTES & CALCULATIONS

WEEKLY MEAL PLANNER

	BREAKFAST	LUNCH	DINNER
MONDAY			

SNACK:

	BREAKFAST	LUNCH	DINNER
TUESDAY			

SNACK:

	BREAKFAST	LUNCH	DINNER
WEDNESDAY			

SNACK:

	BREAKFAST	LUNCH	DINNER
THURSDAY			

SNACK:

	BREAKFAST	LUNCH	DINNER
FRIDAY			

SNACK:

	BREAKFAST	LUNCH	DINNER
SATURDAY			

SNACK:

	BREAKFAST	LUNCH	DINNER
SUNDAY			

SNACK:

NOTES & CALCULATIONS

WEEKLY MEAL PLANNER

	BREAKFAST	LUNCH	DINNER
MONDAY			

SNACK:

	BREAKFAST	LUNCH	DINNER
TUESDAY			

SNACK:

	BREAKFAST	LUNCH	DINNER
WEDNESDAY			

SNACK:

	BREAKFAST	LUNCH	DINNER
THURSDAY			

SNACK:

	BREAKFAST	LUNCH	DINNER
FRIDAY			

SNACK:

	BREAKFAST	LUNCH	DINNER
SATURDAY			

SNACK:

	BREAKFAST	LUNCH	DINNER
SUNDAY			

SNACK:

NOTES & CALCULATIONS

WEEKLY MEAL PLANNER

	BREAKFAST	LUNCH	DINNER
MONDAY			

SNACK:

	BREAKFAST	LUNCH	DINNER
TUESDAY			

SNACK:

	BREAKFAST	LUNCH	DINNER
WEDNESDAY			

SNACK:

	BREAKFAST	LUNCH	DINNER
THURSDAY			

SNACK:

	BREAKFAST	LUNCH	DINNER
FRIDAY			

SNACK:

	BREAKFAST	LUNCH	DINNER
SATURDAY			

SNACK:

	BREAKFAST	LUNCH	DINNER
SUNDAY			

SNACK:

NOTES & CALCULATIONS

WEEKLY MEAL PLANNER

	BREAKFAST	LUNCH	DINNER
MONDAY			

SNACK:

	BREAKFAST	LUNCH	DINNER
TUESDAY			

SNACK:

	BREAKFAST	LUNCH	DINNER
WEDNESDAY			

SNACK:

	BREAKFAST	LUNCH	DINNER
THURSDAY			

SNACK:

	BREAKFAST	LUNCH	DINNER
FRIDAY			

SNACK:

	BREAKFAST	LUNCH	DINNER
SATURDAY			

SNACK:

	BREAKFAST	LUNCH	DINNER
SUNDAY			

SNACK:

NOTES & CALCULATIONS

WEEKLY MEAL PLANNER

	BREAKFAST	LUNCH	DINNER
MONDAY			

SNACK:

	BREAKFAST	LUNCH	DINNER
TUESDAY			

SNACK:

	BREAKFAST	LUNCH	DINNER
WEDNESDAY			

SNACK:

	BREAKFAST	LUNCH	DINNER
THURSDAY			

SNACK:

	BREAKFAST	LUNCH	DINNER
FRIDAY			

SNACK:

	BREAKFAST	LUNCH	DINNER
SATURDAY			

SNACK:

	BREAKFAST	LUNCH	DINNER
SUNDAY			

SNACK:

NOTES & CALCULATIONS

WEEKLY MEAL PLANNER

	BREAKFAST	LUNCH	DINNER
MONDAY			

SNACK:

	BREAKFAST	LUNCH	DINNER
TUESDAY			

SNACK:

	BREAKFAST	LUNCH	DINNER
WEDNESDAY			

SNACK:

	BREAKFAST	LUNCH	DINNER
THURSDAY			

SNACK:

	BREAKFAST	LUNCH	DINNER
FRIDAY			

SNACK:

	BREAKFAST	LUNCH	DINNER
SATURDAY			

SNACK:

	BREAKFAST	LUNCH	DINNER
SUNDAY			

SNACK:

NOTES & CALCULATIONS

WEEKLY MEAL PLANNER

	BREAKFAST	LUNCH	DINNER
MONDAY			

SNACK:

	BREAKFAST	LUNCH	DINNER
TUESDAY			

SNACK:

	BREAKFAST	LUNCH	DINNER
WEDNESDAY			

SNACK:

	BREAKFAST	LUNCH	DINNER
THURSDAY			

SNACK:

	BREAKFAST	LUNCH	DINNER
FRIDAY			

SNACK:

	BREAKFAST	LUNCH	DINNER
SATURDAY			

SNACK:

	BREAKFAST	LUNCH	DINNER
SUNDAY			

SNACK:

NOTES & CALCULATIONS

	BREAKFAST	LUNCH	DINNER
MONDAY			

SNACK:

	BREAKFAST	LUNCH	DINNER
TUESDAY			

SNACK:

	BREAKFAST	LUNCH	DINNER
WEDNESDAY			

SNACK:

	BREAKFAST	LUNCH	DINNER
THURSDAY			

SNACK:

	BREAKFAST	LUNCH	DINNER
FRIDAY			

SNACK:

	BREAKFAST	LUNCH	DINNER
SATURDAY			

SNACK:

	BREAKFAST	LUNCH	DINNER
SUNDAY			

SNACK:

NOTES & CALCULATIONS

WEEKLY MEAL PLANNER

	BREAKFAST	LUNCH	DINNER
MONDAY			

SNACK:

	BREAKFAST	LUNCH	DINNER
TUESDAY			

SNACK:

	BREAKFAST	LUNCH	DINNER
WEDNESDAY			

SNACK:

	BREAKFAST	LUNCH	DINNER
THURSDAY			

SNACK:

	BREAKFAST	LUNCH	DINNER
FRIDAY			

SNACK:

	BREAKFAST	LUNCH	DINNER
SATURDAY			

SNACK:

	BREAKFAST	LUNCH	DINNER
SUNDAY			

SNACK:

NOTES & CALCULATIONS

	BREAKFAST	LUNCH	DINNER
MONDAY			

SNACK:

	BREAKFAST	LUNCH	DINNER
TUESDAY			

SNACK:

	BREAKFAST	LUNCH	DINNER
WEDNESDAY			

SNACK:

	BREAKFAST	LUNCH	DINNER
THURSDAY			

SNACK:

	BREAKFAST	LUNCH	DINNER
FRIDAY			

SNACK:

	BREAKFAST	LUNCH	DINNER
SATURDAY			

SNACK:

	BREAKFAST	LUNCH	DINNER
SUNDAY			

SNACK:

NOTES & CALCULATIONS

WEEKLY MEAL PLANNER

	BREAKFAST	LUNCH	DINNER
MONDAY			

SNACK:

	BREAKFAST	LUNCH	DINNER
TUESDAY			

SNACK:

	BREAKFAST	LUNCH	DINNER
WEDNESDAY			

SNACK:

	BREAKFAST	LUNCH	DINNER
THURSDAY			

SNACK:

DATE:

	BREAKFAST	LUNCH	DINNER
FRIDAY			

SNACK:

	BREAKFAST	LUNCH	DINNER
SATURDAY			

SNACK:

	BREAKFAST	LUNCH	DINNER
SUNDAY			

SNACK:

NOTES & CALCULATIONS

	BREAKFAST	LUNCH	DINNER
MONDAY			

SNACK:

	BREAKFAST	LUNCH	DINNER
TUESDAY			

SNACK:

	BREAKFAST	LUNCH	DINNER
WEDNESDAY			

SNACK:

	BREAKFAST	LUNCH	DINNER
THURSDAY			

SNACK:

	BREAKFAST	LUNCH	DINNER
FRIDAY			

SNACK:

	BREAKFAST	LUNCH	DINNER
SATURDAY			

SNACK:

	BREAKFAST	LUNCH	DINNER
SUNDAY			

SNACK:

NOTES & CALCULATIONS

WEEKLY MEAL PLANNER

	BREAKFAST	LUNCH	DINNER
MONDAY			

SNACK:

	BREAKFAST	LUNCH	DINNER
TUESDAY			

SNACK:

	BREAKFAST	LUNCH	DINNER
WEDNESDAY			

SNACK:

	BREAKFAST	LUNCH	DINNER
THURSDAY			

SNACK:

	BREAKFAST	LUNCH	DINNER
FRIDAY			

SNACK:

	BREAKFAST	LUNCH	DINNER
SATURDAY			

SNACK:

	BREAKFAST	LUNCH	DINNER
SUNDAY			

SNACK:

NOTES & CALCULATIONS

	BREAKFAST	LUNCH	DINNER
MONDAY			

SNACK:

	BREAKFAST	LUNCH	DINNER
TUESDAY			

SNACK:

	BREAKFAST	LUNCH	DINNER
WEDNESDAY			

SNACK:

	BREAKFAST	LUNCH	DINNER
THURSDAY			

SNACK:

	BREAKFAST	LUNCH	DINNER
FRIDAY			

SNACK:

	BREAKFAST	LUNCH	DINNER
SATURDAY			

SNACK:

	BREAKFAST	LUNCH	DINNER
SUNDAY			

SNACK:

NOTES & CALCULATIONS

WEEKLY MEAL PLANNER

	BREAKFAST	LUNCH	DINNER
MONDAY			

SNACK:

	BREAKFAST	LUNCH	DINNER
TUESDAY			

SNACK:

	BREAKFAST	LUNCH	DINNER
WEDNESDAY			

SNACK:

	BREAKFAST	LUNCH	DINNER
THURSDAY			

SNACK:

	BREAKFAST	LUNCH	DINNER
FRIDAY			

SNACK:

	BREAKFAST	LUNCH	DINNER
SATURDAY			

SNACK:

	BREAKFAST	LUNCH	DINNER
SUNDAY			

SNACK:

NOTES & CALCULATIONS

WEEKLY MEAL PLANNER

	BREAKFAST	LUNCH	DINNER
MONDAY			

SNACK:

	BREAKFAST	LUNCH	DINNER
TUESDAY			

SNACK:

	BREAKFAST	LUNCH	DINNER
WEDNESDAY			

SNACK:

	BREAKFAST	LUNCH	DINNER
THURSDAY			

SNACK:

	BREAKFAST	LUNCH	DINNER
FRIDAY			

SNACK:

	BREAKFAST	LUNCH	DINNER
SATURDAY			

SNACK:

	BREAKFAST	LUNCH	DINNER
SUNDAY			

SNACK:

NOTES & CALCULATIONS

WEEKLY MEAL PLANNER

	BREAKFAST	LUNCH	DINNER
MONDAY			

SNACK:

	BREAKFAST	LUNCH	DINNER
TUESDAY			

SNACK:

	BREAKFAST	LUNCH	DINNER
WEDNESDAY			

SNACK:

	BREAKFAST	LUNCH	DINNER
THURSDAY			

SNACK:

	BREAKFAST	LUNCH	DINNER
FRIDAY			

SNACK:

	BREAKFAST	LUNCH	DINNER
SATURDAY			

SNACK:

	BREAKFAST	LUNCH	DINNER
SUNDAY			

SNACK:

NOTES & CALCULATIONS

WEEKLY MEAL PLANNER

	BREAKFAST	LUNCH	DINNER
MONDAY			

SNACK:

	BREAKFAST	LUNCH	DINNER
TUESDAY			

SNACK:

	BREAKFAST	LUNCH	DINNER
WEDNESDAY			

SNACK:

	BREAKFAST	LUNCH	DINNER
THURSDAY			

SNACK:

	BREAKFAST	LUNCH	DINNER
FRIDAY			

SNACK:

	BREAKFAST	LUNCH	DINNER
SATURDAY			

SNACK:

	BREAKFAST	LUNCH	DINNER
SUNDAY			

SNACK:

NOTES & CALCULATIONS

	BREAKFAST	LUNCH	DINNER
MONDAY			

SNACK:

	BREAKFAST	LUNCH	DINNER
TUESDAY			

SNACK:

	BREAKFAST	LUNCH	DINNER
WEDNESDAY			

SNACK:

	BREAKFAST	LUNCH	DINNER
THURSDAY			

SNACK:

	BREAKFAST	LUNCH	DINNER
FRIDAY			

SNACK:

	BREAKFAST	LUNCH	DINNER
SATURDAY			

SNACK:

	BREAKFAST	LUNCH	DINNER
SUNDAY			

SNACK:

NOTES & CALCULATIONS

	BREAKFAST	LUNCH	DINNER
MONDAY			

SNACK:

	BREAKFAST	LUNCH	DINNER
TUESDAY			

SNACK:

	BREAKFAST	LUNCH	DINNER
WEDNESDAY			

SNACK:

	BREAKFAST	LUNCH	DINNER
THURSDAY			

SNACK:

	BREAKFAST	LUNCH	DINNER
FRIDAY			

SNACK:

	BREAKFAST	LUNCH	DINNER
SATURDAY			

SNACK:

	BREAKFAST	LUNCH	DINNER
SUNDAY			

SNACK:

NOTES & CALCULATIONS

	BREAKFAST	LUNCH	DINNER
MONDAY			

SNACK:

	BREAKFAST	LUNCH	DINNER
TUESDAY			

SNACK:

	BREAKFAST	LUNCH	DINNER
WEDNESDAY			

SNACK:

	BREAKFAST	LUNCH	DINNER
THURSDAY			

SNACK:

FRIDAY	BREAKFAST	LUNCH	DINNER

SNACK:

SATURDAY	BREAKFAST	LUNCH	DINNER

SNACK:

SUNDAY	BREAKFAST	LUNCH	DINNER

SNACK:

NOTES & CALCULATIONS

WEEKLY MEAL PLANNER

	BREAKFAST	LUNCH	DINNER
MONDAY			

SNACK:

	BREAKFAST	LUNCH	DINNER
TUESDAY			

SNACK:

	BREAKFAST	LUNCH	DINNER
WEDNESDAY			

SNACK:

	BREAKFAST	LUNCH	DINNER
THURSDAY			

SNACK:

	BREAKFAST	LUNCH	DINNER
FRIDAY			

SNACK:

	BREAKFAST	LUNCH	DINNER
SATURDAY			

SNACK:

	BREAKFAST	LUNCH	DINNER
SUNDAY			

SNACK:

NOTES & CALCULATIONS

	BREAKFAST	LUNCH	DINNER
MONDAY			
SNACK:			

	BREAKFAST	LUNCH	DINNER
TUESDAY			
SNACK:			

	BREAKFAST	LUNCH	DINNER
WEDNESDAY			
SNACK:			

	BREAKFAST	LUNCH	DINNER
THURSDAY			
SNACK:			

	BREAKFAST	LUNCH	DINNER
FRIDAY			

SNACK:

	BREAKFAST	LUNCH	DINNER
SATURDAY			

SNACK:

	BREAKFAST	LUNCH	DINNER
SUNDAY			

SNACK:

NOTES & CALCULATIONS

	BREAKFAST	LUNCH	DINNER
MONDAY			

SNACK:

	BREAKFAST	LUNCH	DINNER
TUESDAY			

SNACK:

	BREAKFAST	LUNCH	DINNER
WEDNESDAY			

SNACK:

	BREAKFAST	LUNCH	DINNER
THURSDAY			

SNACK:

	BREAKFAST	LUNCH	DINNER
FRIDAY			

SNACK:

	BREAKFAST	LUNCH	DINNER
SATURDAY			

SNACK:

	BREAKFAST	LUNCH	DINNER
SUNDAY			

SNACK:

NOTES & CALCULATIONS

WEEKLY MEAL PLANNER

	BREAKFAST	LUNCH	DINNER
MONDAY			

SNACK:

	BREAKFAST	LUNCH	DINNER
TUESDAY			

SNACK:

	BREAKFAST	LUNCH	DINNER
WEDNESDAY			

SNACK:

	BREAKFAST	LUNCH	DINNER
THURSDAY			

SNACK:

	BREAKFAST	LUNCH	DINNER
FRIDAY			

SNACK:

	BREAKFAST	LUNCH	DINNER
SATURDAY			

SNACK:

	BREAKFAST	LUNCH	DINNER
SUNDAY			

SNACK:

NOTES & CALCULATIONS

WEEKLY MEAL PLANNER

	BREAKFAST	LUNCH	DINNER
MONDAY			

SNACK:

	BREAKFAST	LUNCH	DINNER
TUESDAY			

SNACK:

	BREAKFAST	LUNCH	DINNER
WEDNESDAY			

SNACK:

	BREAKFAST	LUNCH	DINNER
THURSDAY			

SNACK:

	BREAKFAST	LUNCH	DINNER
FRIDAY			

SNACK:

	BREAKFAST	LUNCH	DINNER
SATURDAY			

SNACK:

	BREAKFAST	LUNCH	DINNER
SUNDAY			

SNACK:

NOTES & CALCULATIONS

	BREAKFAST	LUNCH	DINNER
MONDAY			

SNACK:

	BREAKFAST	LUNCH	DINNER
TUESDAY			

SNACK:

	BREAKFAST	LUNCH	DINNER
WEDNESDAY			

SNACK:

	BREAKFAST	LUNCH	DINNER
THURSDAY			

SNACK:

	BREAKFAST	LUNCH	DINNER
FRIDAY			

SNACK:

	BREAKFAST	LUNCH	DINNER
SATURDAY			

SNACK:

	BREAKFAST	LUNCH	DINNER
SUNDAY			

SNACK:

NOTES & CALCULATIONS

WEEKLY MEAL PLANNER

	BREAKFAST	LUNCH	DINNER
MONDAY			

SNACK:

	BREAKFAST	LUNCH	DINNER
TUESDAY			

SNACK:

	BREAKFAST	LUNCH	DINNER
WEDNESDAY			

SNACK:

	BREAKFAST	LUNCH	DINNER
THURSDAY			

SNACK:

	BREAKFAST	LUNCH	DINNER
FRIDAY			

SNACK:

	BREAKFAST	LUNCH	DINNER
SATURDAY			

SNACK:

	BREAKFAST	LUNCH	DINNER
SUNDAY			

SNACK:

NOTES & CALCULATIONS

	BREAKFAST	LUNCH	DINNER
MONDAY			

SNACK:

	BREAKFAST	LUNCH	DINNER
TUESDAY			

SNACK:

	BREAKFAST	LUNCH	DINNER
WEDNESDAY			

SNACK:

	BREAKFAST	LUNCH	DINNER
THURSDAY			

SNACK:

	BREAKFAST	LUNCH	DINNER
FRIDAY			

SNACK:

	BREAKFAST	LUNCH	DINNER
SATURDAY			

SNACK:

	BREAKFAST	LUNCH	DINNER
SUNDAY			

SNACK:

NOTES & CALCULATIONS

	BREAKFAST	LUNCH	DINNER
MONDAY			

SNACK:

	BREAKFAST	LUNCH	DINNER
TUESDAY			

SNACK:

	BREAKFAST	LUNCH	DINNER
WEDNESDAY			

SNACK:

	BREAKFAST	LUNCH	DINNER
THURSDAY			

SNACK:

	BREAKFAST	LUNCH	DINNER
FRIDAY			

SNACK:

	BREAKFAST	LUNCH	DINNER
SATURDAY			

SNACK:

	BREAKFAST	LUNCH	DINNER
SUNDAY			

SNACK:

NOTES & CALCULATIONS

WEEKLY MEAL PLANNER

	BREAKFAST	LUNCH	DINNER
MONDAY			

SNACK:

	BREAKFAST	LUNCH	DINNER
TUESDAY			

SNACK:

	BREAKFAST	LUNCH	DINNER
WEDNESDAY			

SNACK:

	BREAKFAST	LUNCH	DINNER
THURSDAY			

SNACK:

	BREAKFAST	LUNCH	DINNER
FRIDAY			

SNACK:

	BREAKFAST	LUNCH	DINNER
SATURDAY			

SNACK:

	BREAKFAST	LUNCH	DINNER
SUNDAY			

SNACK:

NOTES & CALCULATIONS

	BREAKFAST	LUNCH	DINNER
MONDAY			

SNACK:

	BREAKFAST	LUNCH	DINNER
TUESDAY			

SNACK:

	BREAKFAST	LUNCH	DINNER
WEDNESDAY			

SNACK:

	BREAKFAST	LUNCH	DINNER
THURSDAY			

SNACK:

	BREAKFAST	LUNCH	DINNER
FRIDAY			

SNACK:

	BREAKFAST	LUNCH	DINNER
SATURDAY			

SNACK:

	BREAKFAST	LUNCH	DINNER
SUNDAY			

SNACK:

NOTES & CALCULATIONS

WEEKLY MEAL PLANNER

	BREAKFAST	LUNCH	DINNER
MONDAY			

SNACK:

	BREAKFAST	LUNCH	DINNER
TUESDAY			

SNACK:

	BREAKFAST	LUNCH	DINNER
WEDNESDAY			

SNACK:

	BREAKFAST	LUNCH	DINNER
THURSDAY			

SNACK:

	BREAKFAST	LUNCH	DINNER
FRIDAY			

SNACK:

	BREAKFAST	LUNCH	DINNER
SATURDAY			

SNACK:

	BREAKFAST	LUNCH	DINNER
SUNDAY			

SNACK:

NOTES & CALCULATIONS

	BREAKFAST	LUNCH	DINNER
MONDAY			

SNACK:

	BREAKFAST	LUNCH	DINNER
TUESDAY			

SNACK:

	BREAKFAST	LUNCH	DINNER
WEDNESDAY			

SNACK:

	BREAKFAST	LUNCH	DINNER
THURSDAY			

SNACK:

	BREAKFAST	LUNCH	DINNER
FRIDAY			

SNACK:

	BREAKFAST	LUNCH	DINNER
SATURDAY			

SNACK:

	BREAKFAST	LUNCH	DINNER
SUNDAY			

SNACK:

NOTES & CALCULATIONS

	BREAKFAST	LUNCH	DINNER
MONDAY			

SNACK:

	BREAKFAST	LUNCH	DINNER
TUESDAY			

SNACK:

	BREAKFAST	LUNCH	DINNER
WEDNESDAY			

SNACK:

	BREAKFAST	LUNCH	DINNER
THURSDAY			

SNACK:

DATE:

	BREAKFAST	LUNCH	DINNER
FRIDAY			

SNACK:

	BREAKFAST	LUNCH	DINNER
SATURDAY			

SNACK:

	BREAKFAST	LUNCH	DINNER
SUNDAY			

SNACK:

NOTES & CALCULATIONS

MONDAY

	BREAKFAST	LUNCH	DINNER

SNACK:

TUESDAY

	BREAKFAST	LUNCH	DINNER

SNACK:

WEDNESDAY

	BREAKFAST	LUNCH	DINNER

SNACK:

THURSDAY

	BREAKFAST	LUNCH	DINNER

SNACK:

	BREAKFAST	LUNCH	DINNER
FRIDAY			

SNACK:

	BREAKFAST	LUNCH	DINNER
SATURDAY			

SNACK:

	BREAKFAST	LUNCH	DINNER
SUNDAY			

SNACK:

NOTES & CALCULATIONS

WEEKLY MEAL PLANNER

	BREAKFAST	LUNCH	DINNER
MONDAY			

SNACK:

	BREAKFAST	LUNCH	DINNER
TUESDAY			

SNACK:

	BREAKFAST	LUNCH	DINNER
WEDNESDAY			

SNACK:

	BREAKFAST	LUNCH	DINNER
THURSDAY			

SNACK:

FRIDAY	BREAKFAST	LUNCH	DINNER

SNACK:

SATURDAY	BREAKFAST	LUNCH	DINNER

SNACK:

SUNDAY	BREAKFAST	LUNCH	DINNER

SNACK:

NOTES & CALCULATIONS

WEEKLY MEAL PLANNER

	BREAKFAST	LUNCH	DINNER
MONDAY			

SNACK:

	BREAKFAST	LUNCH	DINNER
TUESDAY			

SNACK:

	BREAKFAST	LUNCH	DINNER
WEDNESDAY			

SNACK:

	BREAKFAST	LUNCH	DINNER
THURSDAY			

SNACK:

	BREAKFAST	LUNCH	DINNER
FRIDAY			

SNACK:

	BREAKFAST	LUNCH	DINNER
SATURDAY			

SNACK:

	BREAKFAST	LUNCH	DINNER
SUNDAY			

SNACK:

NOTES & CALCULATIONS

WEEKLY MEAL PLANNER

	BREAKFAST	LUNCH	DINNER
MONDAY			

SNACK:

	BREAKFAST	LUNCH	DINNER
TUESDAY			

SNACK:

	BREAKFAST	LUNCH	DINNER
WEDNESDAY			

SNACK:

	BREAKFAST	LUNCH	DINNER
THURSDAY			

SNACK:

	BREAKFAST	LUNCH	DINNER
FRIDAY			

SNACK:

	BREAKFAST	LUNCH	DINNER
SATURDAY			

SNACK:

	BREAKFAST	LUNCH	DINNER
SUNDAY			

SNACK:

NOTES & CALCULATIONS

	BREAKFAST	LUNCH	DINNER
MONDAY			

SNACK:

	BREAKFAST	LUNCH	DINNER
TUESDAY			

SNACK:

	BREAKFAST	LUNCH	DINNER
WEDNESDAY			

SNACK:

	BREAKFAST	LUNCH	DINNER
THURSDAY			

SNACK:

	BREAKFAST	LUNCH	DINNER
FRIDAY			

SNACK:

	BREAKFAST	LUNCH	DINNER
SATURDAY			

SNACK:

	BREAKFAST	LUNCH	DINNER
SUNDAY			

SNACK:

NOTES & CALCULATIONS

	BREAKFAST	LUNCH	DINNER
MONDAY			

SNACK:

	BREAKFAST	LUNCH	DINNER
TUESDAY			

SNACK:

	BREAKFAST	LUNCH	DINNER
WEDNESDAY			

SNACK:

	BREAKFAST	LUNCH	DINNER
THURSDAY			

SNACK:

	BREAKFAST	LUNCH	DINNER
FRIDAY			

SNACK:

	BREAKFAST	LUNCH	DINNER
SATURDAY			

SNACK:

	BREAKFAST	LUNCH	DINNER
SUNDAY			

SNACK:

NOTES & CALCULATIONS

WEEKLY MEAL PLANNER

MONDAY

	BREAKFAST	LUNCH	DINNER

SNACK:

TUESDAY

	BREAKFAST	LUNCH	DINNER

SNACK:

WEDNESDAY

	BREAKFAST	LUNCH	DINNER

SNACK:

THURSDAY

	BREAKFAST	LUNCH	DINNER

SNACK:

	BREAKFAST	LUNCH	DINNER
FRIDAY			

SNACK:

	BREAKFAST	LUNCH	DINNER
SATURDAY			

SNACK:

	BREAKFAST	LUNCH	DINNER
SUNDAY			

SNACK:

NOTES & CALCULATIONS

WEEKLY MEAL PLANNER

	BREAKFAST	LUNCH	DINNER
MONDAY			

SNACK:

	BREAKFAST	LUNCH	DINNER
TUESDAY			

SNACK:

	BREAKFAST	LUNCH	DINNER
WEDNESDAY			

SNACK:

	BREAKFAST	LUNCH	DINNER
THURSDAY			

SNACK:

DATE:

	BREAKFAST	LUNCH	DINNER
FRIDAY			

SNACK:

	BREAKFAST	LUNCH	DINNER
SATURDAY			

SNACK:

	BREAKFAST	LUNCH	DINNER
SUNDAY			

SNACK:

NOTES & CALCULATIONS

	BREAKFAST	LUNCH	DINNER
MONDAY			

SNACK:

	BREAKFAST	LUNCH	DINNER
TUESDAY			

SNACK:

	BREAKFAST	LUNCH	DINNER
WEDNESDAY			

SNACK:

	BREAKFAST	LUNCH	DINNER
THURSDAY			

SNACK:

	BREAKFAST	LUNCH	DINNER
FRIDAY			

SNACK:

	BREAKFAST	LUNCH	DINNER
SATURDAY			

SNACK:

	BREAKFAST	LUNCH	DINNER
SUNDAY			

SNACK:

NOTES & CALCULATIONS

WEEKLY MEAL PLANNER

	BREAKFAST	LUNCH	DINNER
MONDAY			

SNACK:

	BREAKFAST	LUNCH	DINNER
TUESDAY			

SNACK:

	BREAKFAST	LUNCH	DINNER
WEDNESDAY			

SNACK:

	BREAKFAST	LUNCH	DINNER
THURSDAY			

SNACK:

	BREAKFAST	LUNCH	DINNER
FRIDAY			

SNACK:

	BREAKFAST	LUNCH	DINNER
SATURDAY			

SNACK:

	BREAKFAST	LUNCH	DINNER
SUNDAY			

SNACK:

NOTES & CALCULATIONS

WEEKLY MEAL PLANNER

	BREAKFAST	LUNCH	DINNER
MONDAY			

SNACK:

	BREAKFAST	LUNCH	DINNER
TUESDAY			

SNACK:

	BREAKFAST	LUNCH	DINNER
WEDNESDAY			

SNACK:

	BREAKFAST	LUNCH	DINNER
THURSDAY			

SNACK:

	BREAKFAST	LUNCH	DINNER
FRIDAY			

SNACK:

	BREAKFAST	LUNCH	DINNER
SATURDAY			

SNACK:

	BREAKFAST	LUNCH	DINNER
SUNDAY			

SNACK:

NOTES & CALCULATIONS

WEEKLY MEAL PLANNER

	BREAKFAST	LUNCH	DINNER
MONDAY			

SNACK:

	BREAKFAST	LUNCH	DINNER
TUESDAY			

SNACK:

	BREAKFAST	LUNCH	DINNER
WEDNESDAY			

SNACK:

	BREAKFAST	LUNCH	DINNER
THURSDAY			

SNACK:

	BREAKFAST	LUNCH	DINNER
FRIDAY			

SNACK:

	BREAKFAST	LUNCH	DINNER
SATURDAY			

SNACK:

	BREAKFAST	LUNCH	DINNER
SUNDAY			

SNACK:

NOTES & CALCULATIONS

	BREAKFAST	LUNCH	DINNER
MONDAY			

SNACK:

	BREAKFAST	LUNCH	DINNER
TUESDAY			

SNACK:

	BREAKFAST	LUNCH	DINNER
WEDNESDAY			

SNACK:

	BREAKFAST	LUNCH	DINNER
THURSDAY			

SNACK:

	BREAKFAST	LUNCH	DINNER
FRIDAY			

SNACK:

	BREAKFAST	LUNCH	DINNER
SATURDAY			

SNACK:

	BREAKFAST	LUNCH	DINNER
SUNDAY			

SNACK:

NOTES & CALCULATIONS

WEEKLY MEAL PLANNER

	BREAKFAST	LUNCH	DINNER
MONDAY			

SNACK:

	BREAKFAST	LUNCH	DINNER
TUESDAY			

SNACK:

	BREAKFAST	LUNCH	DINNER
WEDNESDAY			

SNACK:

	BREAKFAST	LUNCH	DINNER
THURSDAY			

SNACK:

DATE:

	BREAKFAST	LUNCH	DINNER
FRIDAY			

SNACK:

	BREAKFAST	LUNCH	DINNER
SATURDAY			

SNACK:

	BREAKFAST	LUNCH	DINNER
SUNDAY			

SNACK:

NOTES & CALCULATIONS

WEEKLY MEAL PLANNER

	BREAKFAST	LUNCH	DINNER
MONDAY			

SNACK:

	BREAKFAST	LUNCH	DINNER
TUESDAY			

SNACK:

	BREAKFAST	LUNCH	DINNER
WEDNESDAY			

SNACK:

	BREAKFAST	LUNCH	DINNER
THURSDAY			

SNACK:

FRIDAY	BREAKFAST	LUNCH	DINNER

SNACK:

SATURDAY	BREAKFAST	LUNCH	DINNER

SNACK:

SUNDAY	BREAKFAST	LUNCH	DINNER

SNACK:

NOTES & CALCULATIONS

WEEKLY MEAL PLANNER

	BREAKFAST	LUNCH	DINNER
MONDAY			

SNACK:

	BREAKFAST	LUNCH	DINNER
TUESDAY			

SNACK:

	BREAKFAST	LUNCH	DINNER
WEDNESDAY			

SNACK:

	BREAKFAST	LUNCH	DINNER
THURSDAY			

SNACK:

	BREAKFAST	LUNCH	DINNER
FRIDAY			

SNACK:

	BREAKFAST	LUNCH	DINNER
SATURDAY			

SNACK:

	BREAKFAST	LUNCH	DINNER
SUNDAY			

SNACK:

NOTES & CALCULATIONS

	BREAKFAST	LUNCH	DINNER
MONDAY			

SNACK:

	BREAKFAST	LUNCH	DINNER
TUESDAY			

SNACK:

	BREAKFAST	LUNCH	DINNER
WEDNESDAY			

SNACK:

	BREAKFAST	LUNCH	DINNER
THURSDAY			

SNACK:

	BREAKFAST	LUNCH	DINNER
FRIDAY			

SNACK:

	BREAKFAST	LUNCH	DINNER
SATURDAY			

SNACK:

	BREAKFAST	LUNCH	DINNER
SUNDAY			

SNACK:

NOTES & CALCULATIONS

WEEKLY MEAL PLANNER

	BREAKFAST	LUNCH	DINNER
MONDAY			

SNACK:

	BREAKFAST	LUNCH	DINNER
TUESDAY			

SNACK:

	BREAKFAST	LUNCH	DINNER
WEDNESDAY			

SNACK:

	BREAKFAST	LUNCH	DINNER
THURSDAY			

SNACK:

FRIDAY	BREAKFAST	LUNCH	DINNER

SNACK:

SATURDAY	BREAKFAST	LUNCH	DINNER

SNACK:

SUNDAY	BREAKFAST	LUNCH	DINNER

SNACK:

NOTES & CALCULATIONS

from seriouseats.com/recipes/2018/03/vegan-fettucine-alfredo
.htm|#recipe — wrapper

RECIPE Vegan Fettucini Alfredo

SERVES	PREP TIME	COOK TIME

INGREDIENTS

1 ½ cups unsweetened, unflavored almond/cashew milk or veg broth

1 lb cauliflower, cored + cut into medium florets

½ cup raw Cashews (203)

2 TBL nutritional yeast

Finely grated zest of ½ lemon

Kosher salt

INSTRUCTIONS

NOTES

RECIPE

SERVES	PREP TIME	COOK TIME

INGREDIENTS

INSTRUCTIONS

NOTES

RECIPE

SERVES	PREP TIME	COOK TIME

INGREDIENTS

INSTRUCTIONS

NOTES

RECIPE

SERVES	PREP TIME	COOK TIME

INGREDIENTS

INSTRUCTIONS

NOTES

RECIPE

SERVES	PREP TIME	COOK TIME

INGREDIENTS

INSTRUCTIONS

NOTES

RECIPE

SERVES	PREP TIME	COOK TIME

INGREDIENTS

INSTRUCTIONS

NOTES

RECIPE

SERVES	PREP TIME	COOK TIME

INGREDIENTS

INSTRUCTIONS

NOTES

RECIPE

SERVES	PREP TIME	COOK TIME

INGREDIENTS

INSTRUCTIONS

NOTES

RECIPE

SERVES	PREP TIME	COOK TIME

INGREDIENTS

INSTRUCTIONS

NOTES

RECIPE

SERVES	PREP TIME	COOK TIME

INGREDIENTS

INSTRUCTIONS

NOTES

RECIPE

SERVES	PREP TIME	COOK TIME

INGREDIENTS

INSTRUCTIONS

NOTES

RECIPE

SERVES	PREP TIME	COOK TIME

INGREDIENTS

INSTRUCTIONS

NOTES

RECIPE

SERVES	PREP TIME	COOK TIME

INGREDIENTS

INSTRUCTIONS

NOTES

RECIPE

SERVES	PREP TIME	COOK TIME

INGREDIENTS

INSTRUCTIONS

NOTES

RECIPE

SERVES	PREP TIME	COOK TIME

INGREDIENTS

INSTRUCTIONS

NOTES

RECIPE

SERVES	PREP TIME	COOK TIME

INGREDIENTS

INSTRUCTIONS

NOTES

PRICE COMPARISONS

ITEM	STORES	PRICES
		$
		$
		$
		$
		$
		$
		$
		$
		$
		$
		$
		$
		$
		$
		$
		$
		$
		$
		$
		$
		$
		$
		$
		$
		$
		$

QTY	NOTES

PRICE COMPARISONS

ITEM	STORES	PRICES
		$
		$
		$
		$
		$
		$
		$
		$
		$
		$
		$
		$
		$
		$
		$
		$
		$
		$
		$
		$
		$
		$
		$
		$
		$
		$
		$
		$

QTY	NOTES

PRICE COMPARISONS

ITEM	STORES	PRICES
		$
		$
		$
		$
		$
		$
		$
		$
		$
		$
		$
		$
		$
		$
		$
		$
		$
		$
		$
		$
		$
		$
		$
		$
		$
		$
		$

QTY	NOTES

PRICE COMPARISONS

ITEM	STORES	PRICES
		$
		$
		$
		$
		$
		$
		$
		$
		$
		$
		$
		$
		$
		$
		$
		$
		$
		$
		$
		$
		$
		$
		$
		$
		$
		$
		$
		$

QTY	NOTES

PRICE COMPARISONS

ITEM	STORES	PRICES
		$
		$
		$
		$
		$
		$
		$
		$
		$
		$
		$
		$
		$
		$
		$
		$
		$
		$
		$
		$
		$
		$
		$
		$
		$

QTY	NOTES

PRICE COMPARISONS

ITEM	STORES	PRICES
		$
		$
		$
		$
		$
		$
		$
		$
		$
		$
		$
		$
		$
		$
		$
		$
		$
		$
		$
		$
		$
		$
		$
		$
		$
		$

QTY	NOTES

PRICE COMPARISONS

ITEM	STORES	PRICES
		$
		$
		$
		$
		$
		$
		$
		$
		$
		$
		$
		$
		$
		$
		$
		$
		$
		$
		$
		$
		$
		$
		$
		$
		$
		$
		$
		$

QTY	NOTES

WEEKLY SHOPPING LIST

DATE:

STORE:

ITEM	QTY
○	
○	
○	
○	
○	
○	
○	
○	
○	
○	
○	
○	
○	
○	
○	
○	
○	
○	
○	
○	
○	
○	
○	
○	

DATE:

STORE:

ITEM	QTY
○	
○	
○	
○	
○	
○	
○	
○	
○	
○	
○	
○	
○	
○	
○	
○	
○	
○	
○	
○	
○	
○	
○	

WEEKLY SHOPPING LIST

DATE:

STORE:

ITEM	QTY
○	
○	
○	
○	
○	
○	
○	
○	
○	
○	
○	
○	
○	
○	
○	
○	
○	
○	
○	
○	
○	
○	
○	
○	

DATE:

STORE:

ITEM	QTY
○	
○	
○	
○	
○	
○	
○	
○	
○	
○	
○	
○	
○	
○	
○	
○	
○	
○	
○	
○	
○	
○	
○	
○	

WEEKLY SHOPPING LIST

DATE:

STORE:

ITEM	QTY

DATE:

STORE:

ITEM	QTY

WEEKLY SHOPPING LIST

DATE:

STORE:

ITEM	QTY
○	
○	
○	
○	
○	
○	
○	
○	
○	
○	
○	
○	
○	
○	
○	
○	
○	
○	
○	
○	
○	
○	
○	
○	
○	
○	

DATE:

STORE:

ITEM	QTY
○	
○	
○	
○	
○	
○	
○	
○	
○	
○	
○	
○	
○	
○	
○	
○	
○	
○	
○	
○	
○	
○	
○	
○	
○	
○	

WEEKLY SHOPPING LIST

DATE:

STORE:

ITEM	QTY

DATE:

STORE:

ITEM	QTY

WEEKLY SHOPPING LIST

DATE:

STORE:

ITEM	QTY
○	
○	
○	
○	
○	
○	
○	
○	
○	
○	
○	
○	
○	
○	
○	
○	
○	
○	
○	
○	
○	
○	
○	
○	

DATE:

STORE:

ITEM	QTY
○	
○	
○	
○	
○	
○	
○	
○	
○	
○	
○	
○	
○	
○	
○	
○	
○	
○	
○	
○	
○	
○	
○	
○	

WEEKLY SHOPPING LIST

DATE:

STORE:

ITEM	QTY

DATE:

STORE:

ITEM	QTY

DATE:

STORE:

ITEM	QTY
○	
○	
○	
○	
○	
○	
○	
○	
○	
○	
○	
○	
○	
○	
○	
○	
○	
○	
○	
○	
○	
○	
○	

DATE:

STORE:

ITEM	QTY
○	
○	
○	
○	
○	
○	
○	
○	
○	
○	
○	
○	
○	
○	
○	
○	
○	
○	
○	
○	
○	
○	
○	

WEEKLY SHOPPING LIST

DATE:

STORE:

ITEM	QTY

DATE:

STORE:

ITEM	QTY

DATE:

STORE:

ITEM	QTY

DATE:

STORE:

ITEM	QTY

WEEKLY SHOPPING LIST

DATE:

STORE:

ITEM	QTY

DATE:

STORE:

ITEM	QTY

WEEKLY SHOPPING LIST

DATE:

STORE:

ITEM	QTY
○	
○	
○	
○	
○	
○	
○	
○	
○	
○	
○	
○	
○	
○	
○	
○	
○	
○	
○	
○	
○	
○	
○	

DATE:

STORE:

ITEM	QTY
○	
○	
○	
○	
○	
○	
○	
○	
○	
○	
○	
○	
○	
○	
○	
○	
○	
○	
○	
○	
○	
○	
○	

WEEKLY SHOPPING LIST

DATE:

STORE:

ITEM	QTY
○	
○	
○	
○	
○	
○	
○	
○	
○	
○	
○	
○	
○	
○	
○	
○	
○	
○	
○	
○	
○	

DATE:

STORE:

ITEM	QTY
○	
○	
○	
○	
○	
○	
○	
○	
○	
○	
○	
○	
○	
○	
○	
○	
○	
○	
○	
○	
○	

WEEKLY SHOPPING LIST

DATE:

STORE:

ITEM	QTY

DATE:

STORE:

ITEM	QTY

WEEKLY SHOPPING LIST

DATE:

STORE:

ITEM	QTY

DATE:

STORE:

ITEM	QTY

DATE:

STORE:

ITEM	QTY

DATE:

STORE:

ITEM	QTY

WEEKLY SHOPPING LIST

DATE:

STORE:

ITEM	QTY

DATE:

STORE:

ITEM	QTY

DATE:

STORE:

ITEM	QTY
○	
○	
○	
○	
○	
○	
○	
○	
○	
○	
○	
○	
○	
○	
○	
○	
○	
○	
○	
○	
○	
○	
○	

DATE:

STORE:

ITEM	QTY
○	
○	
○	
○	
○	
○	
○	
○	
○	
○	
○	
○	
○	
○	
○	
○	
○	
○	
○	
○	
○	
○	
○	

WEEKLY SHOPPING LIST

DATE:

STORE:

ITEM	QTY

DATE:

STORE:

ITEM	QTY

WEEKLY SHOPPING LIST

DATE:

STORE:

ITEM	QTY

DATE:

STORE:

ITEM	QTY

WEEKLY SHOPPING LIST

DATE:

STORE:

ITEM	QTY

DATE:

STORE:

ITEM	QTY

WEEKLY SHOPPING LIST

DATE:

STORE:

ITEM	QTY
○	
○	
○	
○	
○	
○	
○	
○	
○	
○	
○	
○	
○	
○	
○	
○	
○	
○	
○	
○	
○	
○	
○	
○	

DATE:

STORE:

ITEM	QTY
○	
○	
○	
○	
○	
○	
○	
○	
○	
○	
○	
○	
○	
○	
○	
○	
○	
○	
○	
○	
○	
○	
○	
○	

WEEKLY SHOPPING LIST

DATE:

STORE:

ITEM	QTY

DATE:

STORE:

ITEM	QTY

DATE:

STORE:

ITEM	QTY
○	
○	
○	
○	
○	
○	
○	
○	
○	
○	
○	
○	
○	
○	
○	
○	
○	
○	
○	
○	
○	
○	
○	
○	

DATE:

STORE:

ITEM	QTY
○	
○	
○	
○	
○	
○	
○	
○	
○	
○	
○	
○	
○	
○	
○	
○	
○	
○	
○	
○	
○	
○	
○	
○	

WEEKLY SHOPPING LIST

DATE:

STORE:

ITEM	QTY

DATE:

STORE:

ITEM	QTY

DATE:

STORE:

ITEM	QTY
○	
○	
○	
○	
○	
○	
○	
○	
○	
○	
○	
○	
○	
○	
○	
○	
○	
○	
○	
○	
○	
○	
○	
○	
○	

DATE:

STORE:

ITEM	QTY
○	
○	
○	
○	
○	
○	
○	
○	
○	
○	
○	
○	
○	
○	
○	
○	
○	
○	
○	
○	
○	
○	
○	
○	
○	

WEEKLY SHOPPING LIST

DATE:

STORE:

ITEM	QTY

DATE:

STORE:

ITEM	QTY

WEEKLY SHOPPING LIST

DATE:

STORE:

ITEM	QTY

DATE:

STORE:

ITEM	QTY

WEEKLY SHOPPING LIST

DATE:

STORE:

ITEM	QTY

DATE:

STORE:

ITEM	QTY

WEEKLY SHOPPING LIST

DATE:

STORE:

ITEM	QTY
○	
○	
○	
○	
○	
○	
○	
○	
○	
○	
○	
○	
○	
○	
○	
○	
○	
○	
○	
○	
○	
○	
○	

DATE:

STORE:

ITEM	QTY
○	
○	
○	
○	
○	
○	
○	
○	
○	
○	
○	
○	
○	
○	
○	
○	
○	
○	
○	
○	
○	
○	
○	

WEEKLY SHOPPING LIST

DATE:

STORE:

ITEM	QTY
○	
○	
○	
○	
○	
○	
○	
○	
○	
○	
○	
○	
○	
○	
○	
○	
○	
○	
○	
○	
○	
○	
○	

DATE:

STORE:

ITEM	QTY
○	
○	
○	
○	
○	
○	
○	
○	
○	
○	
○	
○	
○	
○	
○	
○	
○	
○	
○	
○	
○	
○	
○	

DATE:

STORE:

ITEM	QTY

DATE:

STORE:

ITEM	QTY

WEEKLY SHOPPING LIST

DATE:

STORE:

ITEM	QTY
○	
○	
○	
○	
○	
○	
○	
○	
○	
○	
○	
○	
○	
○	
○	
○	
○	
○	
○	
○	
○	
○	
○	

DATE:

STORE:

ITEM	QTY
○	
○	
○	
○	
○	
○	
○	
○	
○	
○	
○	
○	
○	
○	
○	
○	
○	
○	
○	
○	
○	
○	
○	

WEEKLY SHOPPING LIST

DATE:

STORE:

ITEM	QTY
○	
○	
○	
○	
○	
○	
○	
○	
○	
○	
○	
○	
○	
○	
○	
○	
○	
○	
○	
○	
○	
○	
○	
○	
○	
○	

DATE:

STORE:

ITEM	QTY
○	
○	
○	
○	
○	
○	
○	
○	
○	
○	
○	
○	
○	
○	
○	
○	
○	
○	
○	
○	
○	
○	
○	
○	
○	
○	

DATE:

STORE:

ITEM	QTY

DATE:

STORE:

ITEM	QTY

WEEKLY SHOPPING LIST

DATE:

STORE:

ITEM	QTY

DATE:

STORE:

ITEM	QTY

WEEKLY SHOPPING LIST

DATE:

STORE:

ITEM	QTY

DATE:

STORE:

ITEM	QTY

WEEKLY SHOPPING LIST

DATE:

STORE:

ITEM	QTY

DATE:

STORE:

ITEM	QTY

WEEKLY SHOPPING LIST

DATE:

STORE:

ITEM	QTY

DATE:

STORE:

ITEM	QTY

WEEKLY SHOPPING LIST

DATE:

STORE:

ITEM	QTY

DATE:

STORE:

ITEM	QTY

WEEKLY SHOPPING LIST

DATE:

STORE:

ITEM	QTY

DATE:

STORE:

ITEM	QTY

DATE:

STORE:

ITEM	QTY

DATE:

STORE:

ITEM	QTY

WEEKLY SHOPPING LIST

DATE:

STORE:

ITEM	QTY

DATE:

STORE:

ITEM	QTY

WEEKLY SHOPPING LIST

DATE:

STORE:

ITEM	QTY

DATE:

STORE:

ITEM	QTY

WEEKLY SHOPPING LIST

DATE:

STORE:

ITEM	QTY

DATE:

STORE:

ITEM	QTY

WEEKLY SHOPPING LIST

DATE:

STORE:

ITEM	QTY

DATE:

STORE:

ITEM	QTY

WEEKLY SHOPPING LIST

DATE:

STORE:

ITEM	QTY

DATE:

STORE:

ITEM	QTY

DATE:

STORE:

ITEM	QTY

DATE:

STORE:

ITEM	QTY

WEEKLY SHOPPING LIST

DATE:

STORE:

ITEM	QTY

DATE:

STORE:

ITEM	QTY

WEEKLY SHOPPING LIST

DATE:

STORE:

ITEM	QTY
○	
○	
○	
○	
○	
○	
○	
○	
○	
○	
○	
○	
○	
○	
○	
○	
○	
○	
○	
○	
○	
○	
○	
○	
○	

DATE:

STORE:

ITEM	QTY
○	
○	
○	
○	
○	
○	
○	
○	
○	
○	
○	
○	
○	
○	
○	
○	
○	
○	
○	
○	
○	
○	
○	
○	
○	

WEEKLY SHOPPING LIST

DATE:

STORE:

ITEM	QTY
○	
○	
○	
○	
○	
○	
○	
○	
○	
○	
○	
○	
○	
○	
○	
○	
○	
○	
○	
○	
○	
○	
○	
○	

DATE:

STORE:

ITEM	QTY
○	
○	
○	
○	
○	
○	
○	
○	
○	
○	
○	
○	
○	
○	
○	
○	
○	
○	
○	
○	
○	

WEEKLY SHOPPING LIST

DATE:

STORE:

ITEM	QTY
○	
○	
○	
○	
○	
○	
○	
○	
○	
○	
○	
○	
○	
○	
○	
○	
○	
○	
○	
○	
○	
○	
○	
○	
○	

DATE:

STORE:

ITEM	QTY
○	
○	
○	
○	
○	
○	
○	
○	
○	
○	
○	
○	
○	
○	
○	
○	
○	
○	
○	
○	
○	
○	
○	
○	
○	

WEEKLY SHOPPING LIST

DATE:

STORE:

ITEM	QTY

DATE:

STORE:

ITEM	QTY

WEEKLY SHOPPING LIST

DATE:

STORE:

ITEM	QTY

DATE:

STORE:

ITEM	QTY

WEEKLY SHOPPING LIST

DATE:

STORE:

ITEM	QTY

DATE:

STORE:

ITEM	QTY

WEEKLY SHOPPING LIST

DATE:

STORE:

ITEM	QTY

DATE:

STORE:

ITEM	QTY

CPSIA information can be obtained
at www.ICGtesting.com
Printed in the USA
BVHW05s0601020818
523221BV00006B/6/P

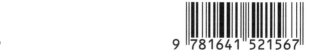

9 781641 521567